Preface

Welcome to "Meal Balancing A Thyroid Diet: Nutritional Strategies for Thyroid Disease. This concise yet informative guide is your companion to understanding the crucial link between nutrition and thyroid health. The thyroid, a tiny gland in the neck with a big impact on our metabolism and energy levels, requires special attention when it comes to our dietary choices.

In this guide, we'll provide you with a solid foundation of knowledge about thyroid diseases and their connection to diet. From the common Hashimoto's thyroiditis to Graves' disease, we'll give you a brief overview of the key thyroid conditions and the role nutrition can play in managing them.

One of the highlights of this guide is the exploration of food sensitivities and their impact on thyroid health. By understanding the interplay between certain foods and thyroid antibodies, you'll gain insights that can help you make smart dietary decisions to support your thyroid.

To keep things practical, we've included a selection of easy-to-follow recipes that align with thyroid-friendly principles. These recipes are designed to not only please your taste buds but also to provide the nutrients that your thyroid craves.

Whether you're seeking a quick reference for thyroid-friendly eating or need a starting point for making informed dietary changes, this guide has you covered. Get ready to unlock the secrets of balancing your meals for better thyroid health – it all begins right here.

Disclaimer from Liability

This book was written and designed by Discover Your Greatest Self℠, under the ownership of Dr. Jasmine Blake Hollywood. By reading this book or viewing any information on the website, social media platforms, in nutrition programs, or services or products, you are agreeing to accept all of this Disclaimer.

The scope of our practice at Discover Your Greatest Self℠ does not include diagnosing or treating medical disease states. Information provided in this book is educational purposes only and is intended as a self-help tool. Health information in this book is not a substitute for physicians' advice, individualized clinical recommendations, or medical diagnoses. You are liable for all risks associated with reliance on this information.

Not all professional nutrition or food expert advice is universally accepted as evidence-based practice. All references listed are either found via research or clinical study resources, and the information in this book is not endorsed by or sponsored by any other organizations. Thus, the views in this book are the author's only and do not reflect the opinion of any professional institution.

You understand that it is your responsibility to furnish the information in this book to a licensed physician before making changes to your lifestyle.If you have a medical concern, are medically ill, or have questions about any medical disease states, speak to your physician for guidance.

Our mission is to support and assist you with reaching your own goals through your personal effort and motivation.

ISBN:978-1-943117-50-5 (Printable Edition)

**Editing by:**
EatItUP™ Editing Team

**Created and Designed by:**
Dr. Jasmine Blake Hollywood

Printed and bound in United States

**Published by:**
Discover Your Greatest Self

True Paleo Inc™
PO Box 130282
Tampa, FL. 33681
www.jasmineblake.com

Table of Contents

# The Guide

**Introduction**

Unlike my usual in-depth explorations, this guide takes a swift route to deliver fundamental insights into the profound relationship between your diet and thyroid health.

Within these pages, you'll find a condensed collection of vital information, distilled into simple and digestible portions. This isn't an encyclopedic textbook, but rather a compass to navigate the complex landscape of thyroid health through nutrition.

Before we proceed, it's important to acknowledge that while this guide offers valuable guidance, seeking the counsel from your healthcare provider or a nutrition practitioner is the wisest choice if you're venturing beyond its scope. Thyroid health is a nuanced domain, and a healthcare professional can provide personalized recommendations tailored to your unique needs.

**Understanding Thyroid Basics**

*The Thyroid's Role in the Body*

The thyroid, a small butterfly-shaped gland nestled in the front of your neck, might be diminutive in size, but its influence on your body is immense. This unassuming gland serves as the conductor of your metabolism, orchestrating the rate at which your body converts food into energy. It does this by producing thyroid hormones – thyroxine (T4) and triiodothyronine (T3) – that have far-reaching effects on various bodily functions.

The thyroid's responsibilities extend beyond metabolism; it influences your body temperature, heart rate, and even plays a role in the development of your nervous system. Think of the thyroid as a maestro, guiding a symphony of bodily processes to ensure harmony and equilibrium.

*Common Thyroid Disorders*

Despite its critical role, the thyroid's delicate balance can be disrupted, leading to various thyroid disorders. Here are a few of the most common ones:

- **Hypothyroidism:** This condition occurs when your thyroid isn't producing enough thyroid hormones. Common symptoms include fatigue, weight gain, sensitivity to cold, and sluggishness.

- **Hyperthyroidism:** The opposite of hypothyroidism, hyperthyroidism involves an overactive thyroid that produces excess thyroid hormones. Symptoms can include rapid heartbeat, weight loss, heat intolerance, and anxiety.
- **Hashimoto's Thyroiditis:** An autoimmune disorder, Hashimoto's leads to inflammation of the thyroid gland, causing hypothyroidism. It's often characterized by the presence of thyroid antibodies.
- **Graves' Disease:** Another autoimmune condition, Graves' disease triggers the overproduction of thyroid hormones, resulting in hyperthyroidism. It can lead to symptoms such as bulging eyes, rapid heartbeat, and weight loss.
- **Goiter:** A goiter is an enlarged thyroid gland that can stem from iodine deficiency, inflammation, or certain thyroid disorders.

Understanding these common thyroid disorders sets the stage for comprehending how dietary choices can influence thyroid health.

**Nutrition and Thyroid Health**

*Impact of Diet on Thyroid Function*

Your diet wields a significant impact on the intricate dance of your thyroid function. What you eat can influence the production, conversion, and utilization of thyroid hormones. Let's take a closer look at how your diet interacts with thyroid health:

Iodine

An essential component of thyroid hormones, iodine is crucial for the thyroid's ability to synthesize T3 and T4. Adequate iodine intake is necessary to maintain healthy thyroid function.

Selenium

This trace mineral plays a vital role in converting T4 (the inactive thyroid hormone) into the active form, T3. It also helps protect the thyroid from oxidative stress and inflammation.

Tyrosine

An amino acid found in protein-rich foods, tyrosine is a building block for thyroid hormones. Including protein in your diet ensures a steady supply of tyrosine for hormone production.

Zinc
This mineral is involved in the production of thyroid hormones and helps regulate their levels in the body.

Vitamin D
Vitamin D deficiency has been linked to thyroid disorders, and maintaining adequate levels of this vitamin is important for overall thyroid health.

Iron
Iron deficiency can impair thyroid function and lead to anemia, which might exacerbate thyroid-related symptoms.

*Essential Nutrients for Thyroid Health*
To promote optimal thyroid function, consider including these nutrient-rich foods in your diet:

- **Seafood:** Rich in iodine and selenium, seafood like fish and shellfish can support thyroid health.
- **Brazil Nuts:** A fantastic source of selenium, just a few nuts can provide your daily requirement.
- **Lean Proteins:** Chicken, turkey, lean meats, and legumes provide tyrosine and other essential amino acids.
- **Leafy Greens:** Spinach, kale, and other greens offer a variety of nutrients including iron.
- **Nuts and Seeds:** Apart from Brazil nuts, other nuts and seeds contribute zinc, magnesium, and healthy fats.
- **Whole Grains:** Whole grains like quinoa provide a range of nutrients including B vitamins.

As you navigate your way through dietary choices, remember that balance is key. An excessive intake of certain nutrients can have adverse effects on thyroid health.

**Food Sensitivities**
*Exploring the Connection*
Unveiling the intricate relationship between food sensitivities and thyroid health opens a window into understanding how what

you eat can influence your thyroid function. While not all thyroid issues are directly linked to food sensitivities, some individuals with autoimmune thyroid disorders, such as Hashimoto's or Graves' disease, may experience exacerbated symptoms due to specific trigger foods.

*Identifying Potential Trigger Foods*
While the specific trigger foods can vary from person to person, some common culprits often associated with thyroid-related sensitivities include:

Gluten
Found in wheat, barley, and rye, gluten can provoke an immune response that might impact thyroid function in susceptible individuals.

Dairy
Some individuals with thyroid disorders might be sensitive to dairy, potentially due to proteins like casein.

Soy
Soy contains compounds called goitrogens that can interfere with thyroid hormone production.

Cruciferous Vegetables
Vegetables like broccoli, cauliflower, and cabbage contain goitrogens as well, which might affect thyroid function when consumed excessively.

Nightshades (Solanaceous Plants)
Certain nightshade vegetables like tomatoes, peppers, and eggplants can potentially trigger inflammation in some individuals.

Artificial Additives
Some artificial additives and preservatives might exacerbate thyroid symptoms in sensitive individuals.

It's important to note that not everyone with a thyroid disorder will experience sensitivities to these foods. However, if you suspect that certain foods might be affecting your thyroid health, keeping a food diary can help identify patterns and make informed dietary adjustments.

*Hidden Triggers*

The journey of uncovering trigger foods is deeply personal, often requiring meticulous observation and experimentation. Consider the case of a client who reported consuming legumes, corn, and potatoes in small amounts with no adverse effects. Yet, after four weeks of avoiding these foods, larger portions triggered episodes of bowel motility issues. This aligns with emerging research that identifies corn as a prominent food sensitivity for individuals with Hashimoto's Thyroiditis (Ostrowska et al., 2021).

Similarly, eggs, a staple in many diets, can elicit unexpected responses. Research has identified eggs as a significant food sensitivity in patients with Hashimoto's Thyroiditis (Ostrowska et al., 2021). One individual reported experiencing slowed bowel motility after consuming eggs, showcasing the intricate interplay between diet and bodily reactions (Whitfield et al. 2022).

Understanding how certain elements interact with the thyroid extends beyond solid foods. Prior alcohol consumption, once considered with a degree of ambivalence, has come under scrutiny. While moderate alcohol consumption was linked to reduced Hashimoto's thyroiditis risk in some studies (Balhara et al., 2013; Effraimidis et al., 2012), recent research points to its potential to suppress T3 and T4 hormone production and exacerbate autoimmunity (Balhara et al., 2013; Caslin et al., 2021). The convergence of findings encourages a cautious approach to alcohol intake, aligning with recommendations to avoid alcoholic beverages due to their high toxic content (Abbott et al., 2019).

*Solanaceous Plants and Thyroid Health*

The discourse surrounding solanaceous plants, commonly referred to as nightshades, is equally fascinating. These plants, including tomatoes, peppers, eggplants, and potatoes, have been the focus of autoimmune thyroid diet protocols. While some diets suggest eliminating them (Abbott et al., 2019), others embrace their inclusion (Caslin et al., 2021).

Research exploring the impact of solanaceous plants on thyroid health presents intriguing findings. While anatabine, a phytochemical found in these plants, has shown potential to ameliorate Hashimoto's Thyroiditis and reduce antibody levels (Schmeltz et al., 2014), contrasting studies highlight minimal sensitivity risks associated with tomatoes in patients with Hashimoto's (Ostrowska et al., 2021). A broader perspective even points to potential benefits, as solanaceous foods like green chilis have been linked to a reduced risk of goiter development, a significant clinical manifestation of Hashimoto's (Jawa et al., 2015).

**Thyroid-Friendly Eating Guidelines**

Navigating the path to thyroid health involves not only selecting the right foods but also crafting meals that work harmoniously with your body's intricate mechanisms. Here, we outline some essential guidelines to help you build meals that support your thyroid function effectively.

*Building Balanced Meals*

Prioritize Nutrient Density

Aim to include a variety of nutrient-dense foods that provide essential vitamins, minerals, and antioxidants. Opt for whole foods like lean proteins, colorful vegetables, whole grains, and healthy fats.

Incorporate Lean Proteins

Proteins such as lean meats, poultry, fish, legumes, and tofu are rich in amino acids like tyrosine, which is vital for thyroid hormone production.

Select Complex Carbohydrates

Opt for whole grains like quinoa, brown rice, and corn. These provide sustained energy and help maintain stable blood sugar levels.

Embrace Healthy Fats

Include sources of healthy fats like avocados, nuts, seeds, and olive oil. These fats are crucial for hormone production and overall well-being.

Fiber-Rich Foods

Fiber supports digestive health and helps regulate blood sugar.

Incorporate vegetables, fruits, and whole grains to boost your fiber intake.

*Portion Control and Timing*
Mindful Portions
Practice portion control to avoid overeating. Listen to your body's signals of hunger and fullness.

Balanced Meals
Aim for balanced meals that include protein, healthy fats, and complex carbohydrates. This combination helps stabilize blood sugar levels and promotes satiety.

Regular Eating Schedule
Strive for regular meal times to maintain consistent energy levels and support your metabolism.

Consider Meal Timing
Some evidence suggests that spreading your meals throughout the day rather than having large gaps between them can help stabilize blood sugar and support thyroid function.

Hydration
Drink adequate water throughout the day. Staying hydrated supports overall bodily functions, including thyroid health.

**Smart Food Choices for Thyroid Health**
When it comes to nourishing your thyroid, making conscious food choices can have a profound impact on your overall well-being. Here, we'll delve into the foods that can support your thyroid health as well as those you might consider limiting.

*Foods to Embrace*

- **Iodine-Rich Foods:** Incorporate iodine-rich options like seaweed, fish (especially cod and tuna), and dairy products (in moderation) to support thyroid hormone synthesis.
- **Selenium Sources:** Include selenium-rich foods like Brazil nuts, seafood, lean meats, and whole grains. Selenium is crucial for thyroid hormone conversion and protection against oxidative stress.
- **Omega-3 Fatty Acids:** Cold-water fatty fish such as

salmon, mackerel, and sardines provide omega-3 fatty acids that help reduce inflammation and support thyroid function.

- **Tyrosine-Containing Foods:** Incorporate lean protein sources like poultry, legumes, and dairy to supply your body with tyrosine, an essential amino acid for thyroid hormone production.
- **Vitamin D Foods:** Fatty fish, fortified dairy products, and exposure to sunlight can help maintain adequate vitamin D levels, which play a role in thyroid health.

*Foods to Limit*

Goitrogenic Foods

These include soy-based products, millet, and certain nuts. While they're generally safe in moderation, excessive consumption might affect thyroid hormone production.

Processed Foods

Limit processed foods high in refined sugars and unhealthy fats. They can contribute to inflammation and disrupt hormone balance.

Sugary Snacks

High sugar intake can lead to blood sugar fluctuations and impact thyroid function. Opt for healthier snack choices like nuts, seeds, and fresh fruits.

Excessive Alcohol

While moderate alcohol consumption might have some benefits, excessive alcohol intake can suppress thyroid hormone production and worsen autoimmune conditions.

Iodine Excess

While iodine is essential for thyroid health, excessive intake from supplements or iodized salt can lead to imbalances. Moderation is key.

Remember, balance is pivotal. Moderation in all aspects of your diet, along with individual considerations, ensures that you're making choices that support your unique thyroid health needs.

**Lifestyle Tips for Supporting Thyroid Health**

Beyond the realm of nutrition, your lifestyle choices play a pivotal role in fostering optimal thyroid function. Let's explore two key aspects – stress management and exercise – that can significantly impact your thyroid health.

*Stress Management*

- **Practice Mindfulness:** Engage in mindfulness techniques like deep breathing, meditation, or yoga. These practices can help reduce stress hormones that might interfere with thyroid function.
- **Prioritize Sleep:** Aim for quality sleep of 7-9 hours per night. Adequate sleep supports overall hormone balance and promotes overall well-being.
- **Limit Stressors:** Identify and manage stressors in your life. Whether it's work-related pressure or personal challenges, finding healthy ways to cope can positively influence your thyroid health.

*Exercise and Thyroid Function*

- **Regular Physical Activity:** Engage in regular exercise to support your metabolism and promote overall well-being. Both aerobic exercises like walking or jogging and strength training can contribute to thyroid health.
- **Avoid Overtraining:** While exercise is beneficial, excessive or intense training can stress the body and potentially impact thyroid function. Listen to your body and strike a balance.
- **Outdoor Activities:** Incorporate outdoor activities to benefit from natural sunlight, which helps regulate circadian rhythms and supports vitamin D synthesis.

Remember that the relationship between lifestyle and thyroid health is multifaceted. By embracing stress-reducing practices and maintaining a balanced exercise routine, you're providing your body with the foundation it needs to thrive.

# The Recipes

**Thyroid-Friendly Grocery Shopping List**

Creating a thyroid-friendly pantry starts with thoughtfully selecting ingredients that support your health goals. Here's a shopping list to guide you as you navigate the aisles of the grocery store:

*Proteins*

- Choose free-range, non-antibiotic, grass-fed or natural-fed meats (poultry, fish, shellfish)
- Include wild-caught fish for omega-3 fatty acids

*Fresh Produce*

- Greens: spinach, spring mix, kale, swiss chard, dandelion, mustard, turnip, collard, romaine
- Colorful vegetables: carrots, peppers (all colors), onions (all types), garlic, celery
- Brassicas: Brussels sprouts, broccoli (all types), cabbage (all varieties)
- Other vegetables: beets, tomatoes (all varieties), chives, peas, cauliflower, squash (all types), Japanese eggplant
- Mushrooms (all varieties), artichoke, asparagus, bok choy, cucumbers, daikon radishes, endive, escarole, fennel, green beans, okra, radicchio
- Add fermented vegetables, sea vegetables, and nutrient-rich microgreens

*Fruits*

- Berries (all types), raw cherries, citrus (all varieties), limited pineapple, pomegranate seeds

*Grains and Seeds*

- Gluten-free whole grains: amaranth and quinoa (small portions, sprinkled on salads)
- Nuts and Seeds: almonds, brazil nuts, chia seeds, coconut, flax seeds, hazelnuts, hemp seeds, macadamias, pecan halves, pine nuts, pumpkin seeds, sesame seeds, sunflower seeds, walnuts
- Homemade nut butters for healthy fats and protein

*Beverages*

- Choose beetroot juice, filtered or mineral water, green

- tea, ginger root, coconut water, or recommended electrolyte formula

*Herbs, Spices, and Condiments*

- Explore a variety of herbs and spices for flavor and health benefits
- Use mustards, vinegars, and approved sauces (refer to the list)

*Dairy Alternatives*

- Opt for nut milks instead of dairy
- Consider coconut milk for cooking and flavor

*Healthy Fats and Oils*

- Use olive oil, avocado oil, flax oil, or coconut oil for cooking and dressing

*Sweets and Treats*

- Choose dark chocolate (70% or higher) for a thyroid-friendly indulgence

*Legumes*

- Include cooked pinto beans, black beans, lentils, edamame, peas, refried beans, and hummus

*Other Essentials*

- Incorporate avocado for healthy fats and nutrients

Remember, this shopping list serves as a foundation for your thyroid-friendly meals. Adapt it to your preferences and dietary needs, and always read labels to ensure the products align with your goals. Your journey to optimal thyroid health involves not only what you eat but also the care you put into selecting your ingredients.

**Quick and Easy Thyroid-Friendly Recipes**

Elevating your thyroid health through nutrition need not be complicated. This section presents a collection of quick and easy recipes designed to infuse your meals with the nutrients your thyroid craves.

*Energizing Breakfasts*

Greek Yogurt Parfait

Layer Greek yogurt with mixed berries, chopped nuts, and a drizzle of honey. This protein-packed breakfast supports your thyroid while kickstarting your day.

Oatmeal Power Bowl

Cook steel-cut oats and top with sliced banana, a sprinkle of chia seeds, and a dollop of almond butter. This fiber-rich breakfast keeps you satisfied and your metabolism engaged.

*Wholesome Lunches and Dinners*

Grilled Salmon Salad

Grill salmon and place it on a bed of mixed greens. Add avocado slices, cherry tomatoes, and a drizzle of olive oil-lemon dressing for a thyroid-nourishing meal.

Quinoa Veggie Stir-Fry

Cook quinoa and stir-fry it with a variety of colorful vegetables like bell peppers, broccoli, and carrots. Toss with sesame oil and a dash of low-sodium soy sauce for a balanced and flavorful dish. Add some gluten-free teriyaki sauce to give it a final touch, and if you like spicy, try szechuan sauce.

*Snacks to Satisfy*

Nut Butter Apple Slices

Spread almond or peanut butter on apple slices for a satisfying snack rich in fiber, healthy fats, and protein.

Trail Mix

Create your own trail mix with a blend of nuts, seeds, dried fruits, and a touch of dark chocolate. This convenient snack provides a mix of nutrients to keep you energized.

Roasted Chickpeas

Toss chickpeas with olive oil and your favorite spices, then roast until crispy. These savory bites offer protein and fiber for sustained energy.

Remember, these recipes are just a starting point. Feel free to modify them according to your preferences and dietary needs. As you embark on your thyroid-friendly culinary journey, consider the guidelines we've discussed so far and the specific foods that align with your health goals.

**Thyroid-Friendly Meal Ideas**

Creating thyroid-friendly meals is a delightful journey of exploring flavors, nutrients, and nourishment. Here are some meal ideas for each week, utilizing the ingredients from your shopping list:

*Week 1*

- Zucchini spaghetti with tomato sauce
- Cabbage and chicken soup with a side salad
- Collards with pork and quinoa
- Squash and cooked Kale with baked fish
  Sauteed leeks, bell Peppers, collards, and quinoa
- Cucumbers and dairy-free salmon spread
- Open-face turkey burger on gluten-free bread with avocado salad

*Week 2*

- Grilled Brussels sprouts with sauteed peppers and onions
- Berries and broth
- Green beans, onions, and lamb
- Cherries, asparagus, and cauliflower
- Beets, garlic, oregano, and sage
- Red bell peppers, broccoli, and beef steak
- Butternut squash, leeks, yellow bell peppers, onions, and garlic

*Week 3*

- Ginger, garlic, and cinnamon-infused chicken with vegetables
- Avocado with cabbage and chicken
- Blueberries, spaghetti squash, and green tea
- Cabbage, carrots, and celery soup with chicken
- Artichokes, mushrooms, celery, flaxseeds, and broth
- Bokchoy, fennel, leeks, citrus, seeds, and broth
- Meat, berries, and spaghetti squash

*Week 4*

- Cod fish with broccoli and carrots

- Chicken with radish leaves and yellow zucchini
- Mushroom and arugula beef stir-fry
- Trout with garlic, onions, and blackberries
- Orange bell peppers, strawberries, yellow zucchini, greens, blueberries, and red onions
- Salmon and purple cabbage
- Pork with berries, romaine, tomatoes, and cucumbers

Use your creativity to adapt these meal ideas to your taste preferences and dietary requirements. With your thyroid-friendly shopping list in hand, these recipes will provide a diverse array of flavors and nutrients to support your journey toward optimal thyroid health. Remember, individual responses can vary, so pay attention to how your body reacts to different ingredients and combinations.

**Thyroid-Friendly Breakfast Recipes**
Kickstart your day with nourishing and flavorful breakfast options that align with your thyroid health goals. Here are some delicious and satisfying recipes that are free from eggs, gluten, wheat, and dairy, along with their replacements.

*A.M. Lovers - Fruit and More*
Breakfast is the cornerstone of your day. Make it your most substantial meal to fuel you until your next one. Morning is when your stomach's acid levels are highest, facilitating better digestion of nutrients.

*Egg White Vegetable Frittata*
Ingredients

- Egg substitutes (approximately 1 cup), beaten
- Sea salt
- Avocado oil
- White onion, chopped
- Cherry tomatoes, cut
- Baby spinach

Directions

- Preheat the oven to 375°F.
- Beat eggs with a little water and sea salt. Set aside.
- Sauté onions and tomatoes in avocado oil until soft. Add spinach and wilt.

- Pour beaten egg substitutes into the skillet, stir to combine vegetables, and cook for about 20 minutes until set.
- Gently loosen edges with a spatula and serve.

*Chia Pomegranate Pudding*
Ingredients

- Chia seeds
- Almond milk
- Pomegranate seeds or berries
- Cinnamon
- Stevia

Directions

- Mix all ingredients in a jar and let it settle for 4 minutes. Stir again until there are no clumps.
- Cover the jar and refrigerate overnight.
- Enjoy in the morning.

*Chocolate Mint Spinach Smoothie*
Ingredients

- Coconut milk
- Cocoa (70% or higher), chopped
- Ice
- Mint leaves
- Baby spinach

Directions

- Blend coconut milk, ice, and mint until smooth.
- Add baby spinach and blend on high speed for approximately 1 minute until well mixed.
- Adjust ice for desired consistency.

*Sausage and Cabbage Soup*
Ingredients

- Turkey or Pork Italian sausage
- Garlic cloves, minced
- Red onion, chopped
- Celery
- Carrots, chopped
- Water
- Tomatoes, chopped

- Baby spinach
- Cabbage

Directions

- Place all ingredients in a large crockpot. Add water to fill it up.
- Cook for 12-24 hours.

*Baked Salmon with Dill*

Ingredients

- Fillets (5 ounces each)
- Dill
- Olive oil
- Sea salt
- Black Pepper
- Brussels sprouts
- Zucchini
- Cherry tomatoes
- Water

Directions

- Preheat oven to 350°F.
- Arrange vegetables in a glass pan. Add salmon fillets on top.
- Season with dill, olive oil, sea salt, and black pepper.
- Add water until the pan is full and cover with foil.
- Bake for about 1 hour or until vegetables are tender.

*Garlic Mashed Cauliflower*

Ingredients

- Cauliflower
- Coconut oil
- Coconut milk
- Sea salt
- Garlic cloves, minced
- Black pepper

Directions

- Steam cauliflower until cooked.
- Blend cauliflower, coconut oil, coconut milk, sea salt, minced garlic, and black pepper until creamy.
- Serve immediately.

*Simple Roasted Butternut Squash*
Ingredients

- Butternut squash
- Olive oil
- Garlic cloves, minced
- Sea salt
- Black pepper

Directions

- Preheat oven to 400°F.
- Toss butternut squash with olive oil, minced garlic, sea salt, and black pepper in a large bowl.
- Spread coated squash on a baking sheet in a single layer.
- Roast at 400°F until tender and lightly browned (about 25–30 minutes).

These breakfast recipes not only cater to your thyroid health but also prioritize flavor and variety. Customize them to your taste preferences and embrace the journey of nourishing yourself with thyroid-friendly meals.

**Thyroid-Friendly Lunch Recipes**
Elevate your midday with these thyroid-friendly lunch recipes, carefully crafted to exclude eggs, gluten, wheat, and dairy, while maintaining the deliciousness and nourishment you deserve.

*P.M. Lovers - Vegetables & More*
Lunch is your nourishing pause in the day. Aim for at least 4 hours after breakfast, ensuring your body receives proper sustenance. With a solid breakfast, your body signals it's time to eat around 3-5 hours later.

*Green Tea Poached Cod*
Ingredients

- Brewed green tea
- Red onion, sliced
- Cherry tomatoes, sliced
- Orange bell pepper, sliced
- Tarragon
- Red pepper flakes
- Sea salt

- Cod fillets
- Black pepper
- Lemon juice, squeezed
- Avocado oil

Directions

- Preheat oven to 350°F.
- Place vegetables, oil, and cod fillets in a glass pan.
- Arrange cod fillets on top of vegetables.
- Season with tarragon, red pepper flakes, sea salt, black pepper, and lemon juice.
- Add brewed green tea until the pan is full, cover with foil.
- Bake for about 1 hour or until vegetables are tender.

*Rib Tips and Vegetables*

Ingredients

- Avocado oil
- Sea salt
- Beef rib tips
- Carrot, sliced
- White onion, chopped
- Yellow pepper, wedged
- Cabbage, chopped
- Dandelion greens, chopped
- Thyme
- Parsley, chopped
- Bay leaf
- Ground cumin
- Garlic cloves, minced
- Water

Directions

- Preheat oven to 350°F.
- Place vegetables, oil, and rib tips in a glass pan.
- Arrange rib tips on top of vegetables.
- Season with thyme, parsley, bay leaf, ground cumin, sea salt, and minced garlic.
- Add water until the pan is full, cover with foil.
- Bake for about 3 hours or until vegetables are tender.

*Mexican Chicken Soup*

Ingredients

- Boneless, skinless chicken breast, cut into ½-inch chunks
- Garlic cloves, minced
- Red onion, chopped
- Red bell pepper, finely chopped
- Tomatoes, finely chopped
- Jalapeño peppers, seeded and finely chopped
- Sea salt
- Black pepper
- Avocados, pits removed, and sliced
- Dairy-free Monterey jack cheese, shredded
- Cilantro, chopped

Directions

- In a large crockpot, combine all ingredients (except vegan cheese and cilantro). Add water to fill the pot.
- Cook for 12-24 hours.
- When done, top with shredded vegan cheese and cilantro.

*Mushroom and Bell Pepper Sauté with Arugula*

Ingredients

- Olive oil, divided
- Mushrooms
- Yellow bell pepper, sliced
- Garlic cloves, minced
- Basil
- Lemon juice, squeezed
- Arugula leaves
- Sea salt

Directions

- Heat 2 tablespoons olive oil in a large skillet over medium heat.
- Sauté mushrooms and bell peppers until tender (7-10 minutes).
- Add garlic and sauté for an additional minute.
- Stir in basil, lemon juice, and arugula, cooking until liquid is reduced by half (about 2 minutes).
- Drizzle remaining 1 tablespoon of olive oil over divided arugula, and top with peppers and mushrooms.

*Walnut-Crusted Fish*

Ingredients

- Flounder fillets
- Almond milk
- Walnuts, chopped
- Sea salt
- Black pepper
- Olive oil
- Lemon juice, squeezed
- Parsley for garnish

Directions

- Rinse fish in cold water and pat dry.
- Dip fish in almond milk, then dredge in chopped walnuts, sea salt, and pepper.
- Cook fish in a skillet with olive oil (3-4 minutes per side) until cooked through.
- Drizzle lemon juice and garnish with parsley.

*Sauteed Vegetables*

Ingredients

- Parsnip, chopped
- Carrot, chopped
- Red onion, cut into ½-inch wedges
- Celery stalks, cut into ¾-inch slices
- Olive oil, divided
- Sea salt
- Black pepper
- Parsley, chopped
- Cilantro, chopped
- Leeks
- Garlic cloves, minced

Directions

- Sautee all vegetables on medium heat until tender.

*Salmon Pecan Cakes*

Ingredients

- Pecans
- Salmon
- Flaxseed meal (replaces eggs)
- Scallions, chopped

- Celery stalk, chopped
- Olive oil
- Lime juice, squeezed
- Sea salt
- Paprika

Directions

- Preheat oven to 350°F.
- Grind pecans to a fine texture in a food processor.
- Combine ground pecans, salmon, flaxseed meal, scallions, celery, olive oil, lime juice, sea salt, and paprika.
- Shape into patties and bake on a lightly oiled tray for about 25-30 minutes.

Explore these thyroid-friendly lunch recipes to nourish your body and indulge your palate. Adjust ingredients according to your preferences and relish the benefits of enjoying a nutrient-packed lunch that supports your thyroid health journey.

**Thyroid-Friendly Dinner Recipes**

Savor the evening with these thyroid-friendly dinner recipes designed to omit eggs, gluten, wheat, and dairy, while embracing delightful flavors and healthful ingredients.

*Late Lovers - Herbs & More*

Dinner marks your final meal of the day, a light affair as your stomach's acid production decreases by this time. Optimal digestion is the goal, so aim for dinner 2 to 3 hours before bedtime.

*Sautéed Sesame Green Beans*

Ingredients

- Green beans
- Olive oil
- Garlic cloves, minced
- Basil
- Sesame seeds
- Sea salt
- Black pepper

Directions

- Steam green beans until fork-tender.
- Heat a skillet over medium, add olive oil and garlic, sauté for 2–3 minutes.
- Add green beans, sauté until warm and coated.
- Toss with basil, sesame seeds, sea salt, and black pepper.

*Baked Lamb Chops with Rosemary*

Ingredients

- Lamb chops (lean)
- Avocado oil
- Rosemary
- Sea salt
- Black Pepper
- Yellow summer squash
- Red onion, sliced
- Leeks, sliced
- Fennel, chopped

Directions

- Preheat oven to 350°F.
- Place vegetables, oil, and lamb in a glass pan.
- Arrange lamb on top of vegetables.
- Season with rosemary, sea salt, and black pepper.
- Add water until the pan is full, cover with foil.
- Bake for about 2.5 hours or until vegetables are tender.

*Cabbage and Beet Greens Soup*

Ingredients

- Yellow onion, coarsely chopped
- Garlic cloves, minced
- Red or yellow bell pepper, chopped

Beet greens

- Cabbage
- Sea salt
- Black pepper
- Parsnip

Directions

- In a large crockpot, combine all ingredients. Add water to fill.
- Cook for 12-24 hours.

*Pinto Bean Vegetable Chili*

Ingredients

- Olive oil
- Pearl onions
- Carrots, diced
- Red bell pepper, chopped
- Garlic cloves, minced
- Jalapeño pepper, seeded and minced
- Chili powder
- Ground cumin
- Dried oregano
- Tomatoes
- Water
- Pinto beans
- Sea salt
- Garnish: Cilantro, chopped; Scallions, chopped

Directions

- In a large crockpot, combine all ingredients. Add water to fill.
- Cook for 12-24 hours.

*Sauteed Kale and Arugula*

Ingredients

- Kale
- Arugula
- Sea salt
- White onion, chopped
- Garlic cloves, minced
- Cherry tomatoes
- Olive oil

Directions

- Sauté vegetables in olive oil over medium heat.
- Add sea salt and garlic, sauté until tender.

*Avocado Lime Soup*

Ingredients

- Lime juice, squeezed
- Cucumber chunks
- Celery
- Romaine lettuce
- Avocado
- Cilantro, chopped
- Water
- Sea salt
- Ground cumin

Directions

- Blend all ingredients until smooth.
- Serve cold, garnished with cilantro.

*Roasted Squash with Greens*

Ingredients

- Spaghetti squash
- Avocado oil
- Lemon juice, squeezed
- Garlic cloves, minced
- Sea salt
- Black pepper
- Rainbow Swiss chard
- Cilantro, chopped
- Leeks, chopped

Directions

- Preheat oven to 400°F.
- Roast spaghetti squash until tender, peel, and gut.
- Whisk together avocado oil, lemon juice, garlic, sea salt, and pepper.
- Pour over Swiss chard, use squash as a base, top with onion and cilantro.

Indulge in these thyroid-friendly dinner recipes to nourish your body, while aligning with your dietary preferences.

Made in the USA
Monee, IL
08 November 2026

67388661R00018